The Atkins Diet

Thomas Curt

Published by RWG Publishing, 2021.

THE ATKINS DIET

First edition. July 15, 2021.

Written by Thomas Curt.

Table of Contents

The Atkins Diet..1

The Atkins and other low carb consumes less calories don't work............3

There's a huge load of new exploration demonstrating the Atkins diet is compelling..5

The new examinations demonstrate that the Atkins diet is sound and doesn't raise cholesterol as recently accepted 7

The Atkins diet will help you keep fat off for great.........................9

Calories don't tally and you can eat however much you need while on the Atkins diet. 11

A fresh out of the plastic new investigation recently demonstrated that the Atkins diet gives you a metabolic benefit so you truly can eat however much you need 13

The Atkins diet causes quicker and more prominent FAT misfortune than ordinary weight control plans.. 15

Carbohydrates make you fat.. 17

Ketosis helps you to have an improved outlook and doesn't influence your presentation 19

Ketogenic consumes less calories (low carb) are the key to fat misfortune 21

The Atkins Diet

Low sugar diets, for example, Atkins have consistently been dubious, yet with the new flood of new exploration and exposure, the contention is currently seething more blazing than any time in recent memory. One feature in the San Francisco Chronicle said that the fight between the low and high carbers had gotten so warmed since mid 2002 that "Blades had been drawn."

From my vantage point (as a wellbeing and wellness proficient down and dirty), it looks more like tanks, ordnance and automatic rifles have been drawn! Deplorably, individuals being harmed the most by these "diet wars" are not the specialists, but rather the weight watchers.

After its unique distribution in 1972, The Atkins Diet was disgorged in 1992 as "Dr. Atkins New Diet Revolution," making another flood of revenue in low sugar slimming down. Then, at that point, in July of 2002, the debate arrived at an untouched high when the New York Times Magazine distributed an exposition by Gary Taubes named, "Imagine a scenario in which everything's been a huge falsehood?" The article proposed that new exploration was currently demonstrating the late Dr. Atkins had been correct from the start.

More exploration in 2003 appeared to prove the Taubes story: Two investigations in the New England Journal of Medicine in May of 2003, and another in June 2003 in the Journal of Clinical Endocrinology and Metabolism, recommended that Atkins was similarly, if not more compelling for weight reduction than ordinary eating regimens – essentially for the time being.

With the distribution of this new data, Atkins allies gloated, "See, I advised you so," while their adversaries terminated back with regards to their high carb, low fat positions. In the mean time, low carb food varieties and enhancements turned into extremely popular, bread and pasta deals experienced a plunge and the wheat business cried the blues.

With contrasts in assessment as inverse as the North and South Poles, it's gotten unendurably befuddling and disappointing to realize which weight reduction strategy is ideal and most secure. At the date of this composition, in late 2003, stoutness has arrived at an unsurpassed high – AGAIN! As per the Journal of the American Medical Association, 64% of Americans are overweight and 31% are stout, it's actually deteriorating.

Clearly, the well known weight reduction strategies today – including the low carb diet – are as yet missing something...but what?

In case you're befuddled by the entire high carb, low carb thing and in case you're disappointed with your efforts to attempt to get in shape and keep it off, then, at that point this might be the main report you will at any point read. In the following couple of moments, you'll find the genuine truth about low carb eats less and a genuine answer for the issue of overabundance muscle versus fat that is delightful in its straightforwardness, yet incredible in viability. Peruse on to become familiar with the 10 Lies about the Atkins diet and reality that will liberate you...

The Atkins and other low carb consumes less calories don't work

Assuming your meaning of what "works" is fast weight reduction, the Atkins Diet DOES work. Ongoing investigations showed that the Atkins Diet causes more noteworthy weight reduction than the American Heart Association-suggested high carb, low fat eating routine. Indeed, for corpulent individuals with problems of starch digestion (hyperinsulinemia, hypoglycemia, and insulin opposition), Atkins-style slims down have been displayed to function admirably.

In any case, in the event that your meaning of what "works" is perpetual fat misfortune, the Atkins diet doesn't passage so well... yet, on the other hand neither do some other eating regimens. It appears to be that regardless of some promising starting triumphs, Atkin's health food nuts actually face similar troubles in keeping off the load as every other person. A portion of similar investigations showing fast weight reduction on Atkins before all else likewise showed considerable weight acquire when the eating regimens finished.

Truly, a developing assortment of proof is mounting that sugar limitation can speed up weight reduction for the time being, yet it still can't seem to be demonstrated that it keeps the fat off over the long haul.

Which approach towards low carb slimming down is best is likewise disputable: Not all low carb eats less carbs are high fat or ketogenic and not all are "super low" in carbs. A low carb diet can be low in carbs and high in fat, it very well may be low in carbs and high in protein, or it very well may be some place in the center

I anticipate that proceeded with exploration will find that moderate carb limitation (particularly in a repetitive design) and cautious choice of sugars, will truth be told help with fat misfortune by means of hormonal control, metabolic proficiency and craving guideline. I accept that neither limit - the seriously confined low carb diet (ketogenic diet) or the extremely high carb, low fat eating routine – will arise the victor.

There's a huge load of new exploration demonstrating the Atkins diet is compelling

In the event that you surf around the Internet for some time looking for "Atkins Diet," you are probably going to see a ton of promotions and news briefs highlighting the new examination "demonstrating" that Atkins is viable.

"New England Journal of Medicine Vindicates Atkins diet." "Studies recommend Atkins diet is protected."

"New exploration challenges 30 years of Nutritional Dogma." Truth is, these features are not giving you the full picture.

Until and except if you have firmly inspected these examinations and the specialist's translation of the outcomes, don't rush to accept the eating routine prattle and tattle.

The overall finish of practically this load of studies is that Atkins IS similarly if not more successful for momentary weight reduction than customary eating regimens. Be that as it may, virtually every one of the specialists additionally close with comments, for example,

"The outcomes are fundamental,"

"The bring home message is that this eating routine merits further examination." "More exploration is required."

Moreover, consider what the Atkin's eating regimen was being contrasted with in these investigations: The customary "food pyramid" diet with 60-65% carbs including a lot of pasta, cereals and bread, correct?

Consider the possibility that the conventional high carb diet isn't right as well.

Try not to discount carb limitation totally, however don't jettison all your carbs yet by the same token...

The new examinations demonstrate that the Atkins diet is sound and doesn't raise cholesterol as recently accepted

In a May of 2003, the aftereffects of a year concentrate on the Atkins diet were accounted for in the New England Journal of Medicine (NEJM). One gathering followed the customary food pyramid with 60% of the calories from sugars while the subsequent gathering followed the Atkins diet.

Following one year, Atkins members had a more noteworthy expansion in the great HDL cholesterol and a bigger drop in fatty oil than the high carb bunch.

The head of the examination, Gary Foster said, "Our underlying discoveries propose that low carb diets might not have the unfriendly impacts we expected."

Standard way of thinking has directed for quite a long time that immersed fat and cholesterol were hazardous and undesirable, adding to coronary illness. This drove most wellbeing experts to denounce low carb slims down that permitted a lot of immersed fat.

This conviction is currently being addressed. Numerous creators, for example, Mary Enig and Uffe Rashnkov have introduced convincing cases that dietary cholesterol and soaked fat don't cause coronary illness. The most recent exploration appears to affirm this. Nonetheless, numerous components influenced the consequences of these new investigations.

In certain examinations, the subjects didn't follow the Atkins Diet to correct details and never entered ketosis, so decisions about immersed fat, dietary cholesterol, ketosis and coronary wellbeing can't be drawn at this point. In different examinations, cholesterol-bringing down drugs were utilized. In still others, a few subjects really showed expansions in all out cholesterol. The individuals who showed upgrades may have recently been on a high refined sugar, high immersed fat eating regimen and dropping the sugar was one positive development. Besides, a portion of the drop in blood cholesterol could be credited to the abatement in body weight.

Plainly, you can't lump all dietary fats into a similar class. Prepared and artificially adjusted trans fats have been denounced by essentially every wellbeing and sustenance master in the world. Different fats, similar to salmon and greasy fish, are among the best and cardio-defensive food sources you can eat. Much proof is showing that sensible measures of normally happening soaked fats, for example, those found in entire eggs and red meat additionally need not be dreaded (particularly without sugars).

Truly, all the data we have accessible as of now shows the "fat fear" and "fat makes you fat" alarm has been unwarranted on the grounds that not all fat is something very similar. Nonetheless, claims that eats less carbs high in by and large and immersed fat are sound and safe for long haul use are as yet untimely.

The Atkins diet will help you keep fat off for great

Dr. Atkins composes that his eating routine "Is so consummately adjusted to use as a lifetime diet that, in contrast to most eating regimens, the weight will not return."

It's a weight reduction maxim that the more outrageous an eating regimen and the quicker the weight reduction, the more troublesome it for the most part is to keep up with the outcomes. Moderate, consistent and adjusted appears to dominate the race with regards to weight control.

Lamentably this isn't what the vast majority need to hear. The four pounds each week and as much as 15 pounds in the initial fourteen days that Atkins guarantees sounds considerably more noteworthy.

There are two things you truly need to think about quick weight reduction:

(1) What sort of weight was lost? What amount of it was muscle versus fat and what amount was water, glycogen and fit tissue?

(2) Are you going to you keep the load off for great?

Most low carbers will not keep the load off for over a year, and many will tumble off the cart well before that.

Keith Ayoob, a representative for the American Dietetic Association, said in an authority ADA explanation about the 2003 NEJM considers: "a year is an equalizer; you hit a stopping point. Your way of life begins to be influenced and you get exhausted. A high dropout rate is an indication that outrageous weight control plans can be hard to keep up with.

Honestly, regardless of Dr. Atkin's cases and the new examination evidently supporting them, we actually don't have a clue what will occur over the long haul. In view of the aftereffects of the new three, six, and year examines, specialists have started to arrange longer preliminaries. One of them will be five years long.

What I trust you will see in long haul contemplates is that Atkins and other low carb slims down, while viable for weight reduction temporarily, will be tracked down not any more powerful for long haul fat misfortune than some other prohibitive eating routine (and that is NOT extremely successful).

Calories don't tally and you can eat however much you need while on the Atkins diet.

Dr. Atkins suggested that calories don't tally and he encouraged his customers to eat however much they need while on his program. Atkins stated, "The supposed calorie hypothesis has been a grindstone around the necks of weight watchers and a hopeless and insult impact on their endeavors to lose."

Here's reality with regards to calories and low carb eats less carbs:

At the point when you go on an exceptionally low carb (ketogenic) diet with more fat, your craving is decreased and you feel more full (since fat is more satisfying than carbs).

Craving control might be a genuine advantage of the Atkins diet, particularly for people who battle with hypoglycemia, yearning and desires. As Dr. Atkins calls attention to, "Our actual desires are difficult to battle."

Nonetheless, this doesn't mean you can eat however much you need. It implies that your yearning might be blunted on Atkin's arrangement, making you naturally eat less without tallying calories or in any event, considering calories.

Individuals on the Atkins diet who get in shape are not eating more than they consume and losing fat despite it. Regardless of whether you tally calories and deliberately eat less than you consume, or you don't tally them and unknowingly eat less than you consume, in any case, the outcome is something similar.

While including calories in the exacting sense is obviously not generally vital, you generally must know about calories and segments. No eating regimen or uncommon blend of food sources can supersede the law of calorie balance.

Any individual who accepts that you can eat however much you need and still get in shape is living in a fantasy world.

A fresh out of the plastic new investigation recently demonstrated that the Atkins diet gives you a metabolic benefit so you truly can eat however much you need

A multi week study led by the Harvard School of Public Health and introduced in October 2003 toward the North American Association for the Study of Obesity found that subjects on a low carb routine lost the same amount of weight as those on a standard high carb, low fat eating regimen.

The stunning part was that the gathering on the Atkins diet could eat 300 a greater number of calories than the gathering eating the ordinary high carb food pyramid diet. This left analysts scratching their heads saying,

"It doesn't bode well... it opposes the laws of thermodynamics."

"A ton of our suspicions about a calorie is a calorie are being tested,"

Sadly, a portion of the Atkins troops rushed to decipher the outcomes as signifying, "See, I revealed to you calories don't check."

In reality, calories do check and the clarification for these outcomes is very basic.

A calorie isn't only a calorie. In the event that all calories were made equivalent, a 2000 calorie diet of Krispy crème doughnuts would have a similar impact as a 2000 calorie diet of chicken bosom and salad vegetables. Do you figure these two eating regimens will have similar consequences for your wellbeing and body arrangement?

Certain food varieties and certain weight control plans DO give you a metabolic benefit. One benefit is the impact of an eating regimen's creation on your chemicals; specifically insulin and glucagon.

leaving a net calorie esteem generously not exactly the aggregate sum of caloric energy that was contained in the food.

For instance, a lean protein food, for example, chicken bosom has a thermic impact of around 20-30%. This implies that for each 100 calories of chicken bosom devoured, the NET energy used by the body is just 70-80 calories. (A few group call this "negative calories.")

Expressed in an unexpected way, this implies you truly CAN get thinner on a more unhealthy admission on the off chance that you eat food varieties with a high thermic impact.

What's particularly intriguing – giving affirmation of the metabolic benefit of a high protein diet – is that the food sources gave in this examination were low carb, yet NOT regular Atkins passage. Rather than heaps of red meat and immersed fat, the subjects in this specific investigation ate generally fish, chicken, mixed greens, vegetables and unsaturated oils.

I believe study's chief, Penelope Green, hit the bullseye when she said, "Perhaps they (the low carb, high protein bunch) caught fire more calories processing their food."

Honestly, not one investigation has at any point demonstrated that you can "eat however much you need" on Atkins or any eating regimen. In any event, when an eating regimen gives a metabolic benefit, AFTER that benefit is figured in and you take a gander at NET calorie use, you are still left with the calories in versus calories out condition.

The Atkins diet causes quicker and more prominent FAT misfortune than ordinary weight control plans

Most wellbeing, clinical and sustenance associations suggest that you get in shape (muscle to fat ratio) at a pace of close to 2 pounds each week. In his book, Dr. Atkins says that the normal weight reduction in the initial fourteen days on his arrangement is 8 to 15 pounds.

In the same way as other eating regimens, Atkins overemphasizes complete weight reduction (and speedy weight reduction), while not focusing on sufficient the distinction between body weight, body water, muscle to fat ratio and slender weight.

Truly, low carb slims down unquestionably cause more prominent weight reduction, particularly in the underlying stages. Be that as it may, this is for the most part because of a huge drop in water weight and glycogen (put away starch), not really expanded fat misfortune.

Weight reduction is some unacceptable objective! Your objective ought to be lasting fat misfortune and you ought to quantify and following your muscle versus fat ratio and fit weight consistently.

Try not to boast over enormous, quick "weight losses"... it very well may be generally water and muscle.

Carbohydrates make you fat

Dr. Atkins composed, and I quote, "Sugars are the very food that makes you fat." He additionally stated, "Diets high in starches are definitely what most overweight individuals don't require and can't get thin on."

These are deluding proclamations of misleading statement.

The "carbs make you fat" legend is presumably the most inescapable and harming lie about weight control at any point told. It's created huge turmoil and disappointment to effectively confounded and baffled calorie counters.

In the first place, zeroing in basically on any macronutrient (protein, carbs or fat) or macronutrient proportion ought to be optional to energy balance. What makes you fat is eating such a large number of calories.

Honestly, you can't fault all "starches" collectively for why we are getting fatter. What sort of starches would we say we are discussing? There are acceptable carbs and awful carbs. The "awful" carbs are the refined ones; white flour and white sugar items like white bread, white pasta, sugar improved cereals, candy and soda pops.

To keep away from disarray, I would propose always failing to utilize "starch" without putting the descriptive word "refined" or "regular" before it.

Unexpectedly, Dr. Atkins makes this qualification in his book, yet he actually decided to suggest expulsion of practically ALL carbs during the enlistment and weight reduction periods of his eating routine - even the great carbs that are demonstrated solid. This makes quick weight reduction and the presence of an enormously fruitful eating regimen directly right off the bat.

Once more, the genuine inquiries are: What sort of weight was lost and would you be able to keep the load off for great?

A sound, viable fat consuming eating regimen ought to be focused on normal food sources – and for a great many people, that incorporates regular carbs with some restraint - not the complete evacuation and belittling, all things considered.

Ketosis helps you to have an improved outlook and doesn't influence your presentation

Your body is a striking machine that is completely equipped for adjusting to whatever fuel is given in power. You can consume protein, fat, or carbs for energy. Nonetheless, carbs are your body's liked – and generally effective - fuel hotspot for enthusiastic actual work.

Numerous low carbers accept that fat is a more productive fuel source than starches, however this isn't accurate. Fat is definitely not a more effective fuel source, it's anything but a more thought fuel source.

Since the fuel for strong withdrawal is carbs (glycogen) a high fat, low carb diet isn't the best way to deal with fat misfortune for competitors, weight lifters or exceptionally dynamic people. These eating regimens basically don't uphold extreme focus preparing.

Exceptionally low carb diets may be proper for the inactive, seriously overweight, or those with muscular conditions that forestall any activity. It appears to be that ketogenic eats less drop weight even with practically no activity (albeit the weight will not be unadulterated fat and you may not keep it off). Some Atkins weight watchers even report feeling more enthusiastic subsequent to adjusting to the low carbs and higher fat. It's conceivable, in any case, that the majority of them were generally dormant. Low carbs and high movement turn out poorly together.

Honestly, a more adjusted eating routine of normal food sources joined with practice is a vastly improved approach to take off unadulterated fat for great.

Any individual who CAN exercise SHOULD work out! Of the two strategies for making a calorie shortage – consuming more, or eating less – the previous is the unrivaled strategy with far less drawbacks. Any fat misfortune program that doesn't make practice the focal point is at last bound for disappointment.

Ketogenic consumes less calories (low carb) are the key to fat misfortune

The expression "low carb" is utilized comprehensively. To nearly, an eating routine like the Zone, which comprises of 40% carbs is "low carbs." To others "low carb" is more limit. A ketogenic diet is a VERY low carb diet, generally between 40-70 grams of carbs each day or less. The enlistment period of the Atkins diet is restricted to just 20 grams each day.

Since they permit for all intents and purposes no starch, Ketogenic consumes less calories, by definition, are very severe and healthfully lopsided. It's a permanent law that the more "outrageous" a nourishment program is, the more noteworthy the results will be and the more troublesome the eating regimen will be to remain on.

Dr. Atkins guaranteed, "Ketosis is the distinct advantage of very successful consuming less calories."

Honestly, while some new investigations have proposed low carb eats less manage job, not a solitary report has demonstrated that it's important to limit carbs so seriously that you go into ketosis.

The advantages of decreased carbs and more protein incorporate a higher thermic impact, hunger guideline and hormonal control. What the low carb people don't need you to know is that a moderate decrease in carbs (as well as evacuation of handled carbs) is frequently everything necessary to get these advantages, while being a lot simpler to keep up with for the long stretch.

So if ketogenic and exceptionally low carb counts calories aren't the most ideal approach to accomplish lasting fat misfortune, then, at that point what is the most ideal way???

Dr Atkins made numerous astounding focuses about weight control in his book. He stood up on the disasters of prepared sugars. He recognized sugar affectability and hyperinsulinemia as contributing variables in corpulence. He talked about the metabolic benefit of high protein. He brought up that there may not be an immediate coordinated relationship between's soaked fat, dietary cholesterol and coronary illness.

The truth of the matter is, Dr. Atkins – shockingly – had found some significant realities about weight control, and dared to distribute and remain by them some time before any other individual did. Eventually, lamentably, he reached some sketchy determinations from this data and, as so numerous other eating routine masters, he left out some enormous and significant pieces to the riddle.

On the off chance that lasting fat misfortune were just about as straightforward as eliminating sugars from your eating routine, why has corpulence flooded to an all-new high in 2003 and for what reason are there so numerous Atkins disappointments?

Could it be conceivable that the ordinary high carb, low fat food pyramid approach and the Atkins diet approach have BOTH come up short, and that the ideal eating routine for perpetual fat misfortune is some place in the center?

Could it be conceivable that eating less junk food is the most awful approach to lose muscle versus fat and that the appropriate kind of activity program joined with a more adjusted way to deal with nourishment is the appropriate response?

Probably the greatest mistake weight reduction searchers make today is to acknowledge one way of thinking totally or reject it's anything but, a side and "waging war" to guard their situation without thinking about the other options. A large portion of the weight reduction methods of reasoning being advanced today contain admirable sentiments, yet in general, are a complete mixed bag of truth, misleading statements and untruths.

That is the reason, for more than 20 years, I have in a real sense transformed myself into a human guinea pig as I continued looking for a reasonable and sound strategy for perpetual fat misfortune. I concentrated and afterward by and by tried the ketogenic diet, the high carb diet, low fat eating routine and virtually every other eating regimen in the middle. I discovered valid statements and awful focuses in every one of them, a large number of which I have effectively uncovered to you in this report.

I then, at that point arranged every one of the positive marks of each fat misfortune strategy into an organized organization, while disposing of the relative multitude of negatives. What arose was absolutely wonderful: An all-normal framework that has permitted me to top at a muscle to fat ratio level of 3.4% and to keep up with my muscle versus fat at 9% or less lasting through the year... without drugs, outrageous weight control plans, or superfluous enhancements. It's worked for a huge number of others as well.

Don't miss out!

Visit the website below and you can sign up to receive emails whenever Thomas Curt publishes a new book. There's no charge and no obligation.

https://books2read.com/r/B-A-JPNP-LCMQB

BOOKS 2 READ

Connecting independent readers to independent writers.

About the Publisher

Accepting manuscripts in the most categories. We love to help people get their words available to the world.

Revival Waves of Glory focus is to provide more options to be published. We do traditional paperbacks, hardcovers, audio books and ebooks all over the world. A traditional royalty-based publisher that offers self-publishing options, Revival Waves provides a very author friendly and transparent publishing process, with President Bill Vincent involved in the full process of your book. Send us your manuscript and we will contact you as soon as possible.

Contact: Bill Vincent at rwgpublishing@yahoo.com www.rwgpublishing.com